TIE ONE ON

A Head-Scarf Tying Guide for Chemotherapy Patients

by

Pamela Phillips

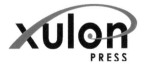

Tie One On
A Head-Scarf Tying Guide for Chemotherapy Patients
by Pamela Phillips

Printed in the United States of America

ISBN 9781613794920

Bible quotations are taken from
THE HOLY BIBLE, NEW INTERNATIONAL VERSION.
Copyright © 1973, 1976, 1984 by International Bible Society.
Used by permission of Zondervan Bible Publishers.

www.xulonpress.com

Dedication

This book is dedicated to all of my cancer sisters.

Psalm 147:3
He heals the brokenhearted and binds up their wounds.

Jeremiah 29:11
"For I know the plans I have for you," declares the Lord,
"Plans to prosper you and not to harm you,
Plans to give you hope and a future."

Table of Contents

Foreword

I remember the day that Pamela Phillips and I met. Pamela already knew that she had a terrible disease ~ "Cancer". She understood that the cancer was serious and that she would need aggressive treatment. She experienced the anxiety and the fear of the unknown as does every woman who comes to my office with a scary diagnosis, without a plan. During the course of our initial appointment, not only did Pamela develop an understanding of what the diagnosis meant, she wanted to move forward as quickly as possible. We decided to proceed with neoadjuvant chemotherapy followed by surgery three months later. Within three hours of our first meeting, Pamela was in our chemotherapy infusion suite actively treating her cancer.

Her proactive approach has been inspiring. She has always wanted to be in control ~ by being one step ahead ~ at least as far as knowing what to expect with her disease progression. I see her sharing that spirit through her book ~ by encouraging women to take control of the side effect of hair loss and by creating their own individual style, while also stressing the importance of comfort and self care. She eloquently shares her life story, starting as a 5 year old who was able to take care of herself, and continues through the present day as she takes on the challenges of continued treatment of her primary peritoneal carcinoma.

She continually provides strength and hope for each woman who understands what it means to lose her hair as part of her journey through cancer. It has been my privilege to be a part of Pamela's life.

Lisa McCluskey, M.D.
Gynecological Oncologist
Northwest Cancer Specialists
Portland, Oregon

I was just thinking what a wonderful gift it would be for someone who is about to lose their hair to receive from a friend a copy of your book wrapped in a couple of beautiful scarves. I can't think of anything that would be more uplifting.

Dee Cohler, Editor

As a woman who did not like wearing wigs because they are itchy, hot and uncomfortable, I wore bandanas because they were available and easy to put on. I had no idea that scarves could be made to look so fashionable, and that learning how to tie a scarf is something that any woman can learn with the right teacher.

This book is a gift for women who would like to look their best during chemotherapy without having to wear a wig.

Diane Rader O'Connor
7 year Ovarian Cancer Survivor
President
Ovarian Cancer Alliance of Oregon and SW Washington

"What an amazing gift you are giving to other women."

Acknowledgements

First and foremost, this book would not have been as useful for the reader without the talents of my photographer, Andrew Creasy. Andrew did a fantastic job on these beautiful photographs and his enthusiasm for the project matched mine, thereby encouraging me on this vision.

I also must thank P.E.O. Chapter BG for being the conduit through which Andrew and I met. Crystal Huffman and especially Martha Shepherd were responsible for this meeting of talents.

And what would photographs be without beautiful models? Thank you, Brenda and Marcy. These two ovarian cancer survivors showed their strength and resilience in our long photo sessions ~ always giving their best for this undertaking. Each of them exhibited strength of character and beautiful confidence in their new cancer-fighting bodies. I am grateful to them for their generosity, not only of time, but also for the generosity of their beautiful spirits.

My editor, Dee Cohler, made necessary corrections, suggested additions, formatted the manuscript and helped my words become press worthy. Dee initially offered to help when I couldn't type because of a shoulder injury. She was indeed a Godsend to me arriving on the scene at the perfect time. She immediately became my primary editor and we spent a week on the phone revising the manuscript multiple times (at least 50) making sure it was saying to you, the reader, what I wanted it to say. Thank you, Dee, my soon-to-be Sister; I know that I could not have done this without your loving help and considerable talents.

Special loving thanks go to Heather Schlegel, Shanon Schlegel, Sue Bouris and Eleanor Boyd for their welcome suggestions, corrections and valued friendships. I am so blessed to have each of you in my life.

Big thanks go to my precious Aedyn for giving Nonni the will to live and for being the best medicine I could ever have.

To my son, Chad Schlegel, who has stood by me and helped me to make sense of the confusing maze that is cancer, thank you.

I also want to thank my Doctor, Lisa McCluskey, M.D. Her encouraging, positive attitude throughout the course of this disease has coincided with my own. I trust her with my life. I also want to thank her for reviewing my book and for her kind comments.

A special thank you must go to the Elegant Gals of P.E.O. Chapter EG. They immediately came and stood beside me and enfolded me in their loving ways from the beginning of my diagnosis.

Heidi Simonet, the Northwest District Manager of Chico's Women's Stores, provided the mannequin and some of the scarves used in the photographs. Her enthusiasm about this project was an encouragement to me when I needed it. Thank you, Heidi.

The scarves featured in this book are special loving gifts from Eleanor Boyd, Glenna Groendyke, Bob and Winni Page, and Heather Schlegel as well as the personal scarves of Brenda McGowan and the author. Their beautiful colors enhanced the visuals that you see.

The author's cover photo was taken by Duane Stork of Atlanta at the 2010 Ovarian Cancer National Alliance Conference in Washington, D.C.

I would like to thank the prayer warriors, my friends who prayed for me when I was unable to do so myself. You have enabled me to have the strength, courage and focus to complete the tasks that I must.

Interior Photographs
Generously Provided
by
Andrew Creasy
creasya@gmail.com

Introduction

After a year of chemotherapy and 16 months of wearing headscarves, I have learned many different ways to cover my head. During that time, when I had enough energy to go out shopping, strangers would frequently stop me and comment on how beautiful my turban-tied scarf looked. I didn't think too much of it until the women at my support group asked me to demonstrate how I had tied my scarf. It was then that I decided that perhaps an instructional book would be helpful to those of us who have chemotherapy and its unwanted side effects as an ongoing part of our lives.

It is difficult for anyone to lose their hair. Even though men are more likely to be prepared for the balding process, many of them still experience a loss of self-confidence. It is a much more devastating experience when a woman loses her hair, especially when it is accompanied by the unwelcome news that you have a life-threatening illness such as cancer.

This issue is more profound in women who have very beautiful tresses. I was not one of those women. Whatever my gifts may be, having gorgeous hair was not one of them, and so for me the thought of losing my hair was actually a non-issue. Or so I thought until the night that it actually fell out. Yes, I cried. For whatever flaws I may have, this one could not be covered up with make-up. It was out there for the entire world to see and wonder about. Now I had to figure out who I was all over again. Even without the hair loss, with the diagnosis of cancer, this re-evaluation would have been necessary.

I did possess a skill and a confidence that had been growing within me since I was five years old. I knew that I could tie a scarf on my head. And so I did.

I hope that this book will give you confidence in creating a beautiful way to wear your chemotherapy side-effects with flair and grace.

Prologue

〜

After retiring as a Flight Attendant with a major United States carrier, I decided that I had many good stories that I wanted to tell. My daughter, Heather Schlegel, helped me start my blog, www.pdxfirefly.com, where I write under the name of Portland Firefly. This prologue is one of those stories and I hope you enjoy it.

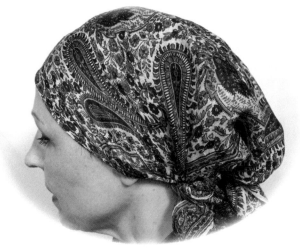

My Childhood Scarf

It was early spring in sunny Southern California and a stray kitty found its way into my little arms. I didn't have a kitty cat and I really wanted this one…so I decided to make this mangy stray my own. Doing what most little 5-year-old girls would do, I began to comb its fur. I guess my bangs got in the way and I decided to comb my hair as well, taking turns combing first the kitty's fur, then my own hair. I remember it vividly to this day; I was wearing a pastel plaid dress while playing with this stray kitty on the warm sunlit driveway.

The next thing I remember is my Mother all dressed up in her pretty dress and heels taking me to the doctor's office. You see, I had contracted a highly-contagious disease ~ ringworm ~ from this kitty that I loved so much.

The then-required treatment was to shave the person's head and keep it covered for many months until all the infected hairs were gone and the new hair had grown in. Since my Mother resisted shaving my head and fought to keep some of my hair, the doctor instructed her in an unusual protocol. She cut my hair very short all over, almost shaving several of the infected areas, while painfully pulling out any stray infected hairs that she could see. She painstakingly plucked them out with tweezers while I was sleeping so I wouldn't scream and run away. My now very short hair with patches of baldness throughout was covered with a beautiful silk scarf my Father had imported from India.

Because of the contagious nature of ringworm, I had to keep my head covered all the time. This continued for many months. My constantly wearing a scarf in school must have been a curiosity to the other children. I remember the pain, the embarrassment, the humiliation and the confusion (were there jeers and taunting, too?) when a boy in my class pulled the scarf off of my head. Did he intend to be mean, or was he just curious? Even today I remember the uncertain, pained look on my teacher's face. I see tears in her eyes matching my own as she views my ugly sparse hair for the first time. Realizing what has happened, she moves all the children to the other side of the bank of painting easels ~ to give me some privacy. Her clumsiness and embarrassment for me are evident as she quickly attempts to re-tie the beautiful silk scarf on my tiny sobbing head. She tries several times. It doesn't stay put. I remember her asking, "Is this the way your Mommy ties it?"

This humiliated 5-year-old knows that the scarf isn't tied correctly. Somehow I get brave and strong through my tears and courageously say, "I can do it. I know how to tie it myself." I know that I can. And I tie the scarf. But it is not as tight as my Mommy ties it every morning for an active 5-year-old. During the rest of the day, my scarf keeps slipping and I have to re-tie it many times. I do make it through the rest of the day, and I return to school the next morning and every morning after that.

I had no way of knowing that the eventual consequences of this event would probably affect me for the rest of my life.

I don't really like cats now.

And I know how to tie scarves really well!

Chapter One

Why Wear a Scarf?

❧

This little book was born out of necessity. Diagnosed with Primary Peritoneal Carcinoma (the rare aggressive sister of Ovarian Cancer), I lost all of my hair two and a half weeks after my first chemo infusion.

Yes, I have wigs, but they have their drawbacks. Some women find them itchy as well as hot, and they tend to shift on your head. I can only stand to wear one for a few hours at a time and only on special occasions. I think a wig gives me what others consider a more normal appearance, and hopefully, for their sake, they can forget that I am sick, at least for a short while. Usually, I will wear a wig for the people that will be looking at me rather than wearing it for myself. I have come to the conclusion that when I wear a scarf, it is a reminder to those looking at me that, yes, I do have cancer.

I recall a delicious dinner with my brother and his wife. I sat at their table wearing the comfortable scarf that I had been wearing all day. I could see the pain in my brother's eyes as he looked at me, trying to get used to my new turbaned look, trying to not think of what it might eventually mean. I quickly excused myself and returned wearing my complimentary American Cancer Society wig that I had brought along on this short trip. He commented that the wig looked really cute and he liked it a lot, so I wore it for them the rest of the night.

That being said, I prefer wearing scarves. They are so comfortable and soft that my scarf can be worn for 10 - 12 hours a day without feeling uncomfortable. With a wig I can hardly wait to rip it off my head. And I usually do so in my car, where I have a little soft knitted cap waiting to keep my head warm.

One big advantage of scarf-wearing is that it is a non-verbal clue to some people that you may not have the energy that most people have. I have found that when I wear a scarf, others often offer to help me, and the help is usually needed and much appreciated.

Chapter Two

Let's Go Scarf Shopping!

W hat is the best type of scarf to use? I prefer scarves that have a color scheme that will enhance a particular outfit I might choose to wear. When shopping for color, remember that you will want a scarf to coordinate with your outfit, not necessarily to match it exactly. Your scarf will be more interesting if it has more than one color in it or more than one shade of the same color. For best results, try to have at least one color in your scarf that is close to the predominant color in your outfit. Another variety of scarf to search for when shopping is one having two colors that if combined together might be the same shade as the top or bottom you will be wearing.

It is not necessary to match the intensity of the colors in your scarf to the intensity of your outfit, although it is usually a good idea to do so. Again, you are striving for the overall effect of how your tied scarf enhances and individualizes your outfit. Use a full-length mirror to determine this. A bold scarf may add just the right punch of color you need to spice up what could be a drab outfit; the reverse is also true, a softer colored scarf may help to tone down an otherwise too bright outfit.

For most occasions, you want to avoid scarves that have several unrelated bold colors in them or one that is too boldly striped. The exception is if you are wearing a monochromatic outfit and you want to draw attention to your scarf. Then you may want to choose a scarf with a bold coloration. Make sure that these colors are flattering to your skin tone. You do want to try to look your best, even while you are still in chemotherapy.

If you are familiar with the colors in your closet, you already have a good idea of the specific colorations you should want in your scarves. I have found that the very first scarf that catches my eye when I walk into a store is usually the one I end up purchasing. The reason for this is that we are drawn to the colors that please us, and hopefully you feel and look good in those colors.

If you have ever had your colors done and you know what colors complement your skin tone, then buy scarves in those colors, because they probably will harmonize with your existing wardrobe. If you know what season you are, then stick with those colors. I am a winter, as are 75% of women, most strawberry blonds are spring, auburn-haired beauties are usually autumns, and then there are the delicate blonds of summer. Thinking of the colors that predominate in nature during each season will guide you toward choosing the best colors for your individual season.

Some of my favorite scarves are umbra ~ which means that they are several shades of one color. Once twisted and tied in a turban, the effect is stunning. My favorite goes from dark teal to a lighter aqua. Teal is, after all, the color for ovarian cancer and is a color that most women can wear easily. Other scarves may have a subtle stripe or a ribbon of metallic thread running through them, and many pashminas are designed with a beautiful paisley pattern. The variety of colors and patterns will make your scarf very interesting once it is twisted and tied atop your head. One of my favorite scarves has a very dark navy blue stripe running through it and this one presents a very good combination with my dark blue jeans and a top of any color.

When scarf shopping, I prefer to purchase the long rectangular scarves and pashminas that are so fashionable now. These long scarves will give you the best options for wrapping and tying. Readily available at reasonable prices in many stores, they are offered in a variety of fabrics and colors. And…after your hair grows back, you can wear them as an accessory. I have included a section on various ways to style your scarves after your hair grows back.

Look for a scarf that is not sheer. A sheer scarf will not hide your baldness. If you find a sheer scarf that you absolutely love, buy it. I'll tell you how to wear it in a later chapter.

More often than not, you will find yourself wanting to wear the scarves that feel the softest; so touch the scarf you are about to buy. If it feels "Oh so soft!" between your fingers, then it will become one of your favorites because it will feel soft and comfortable on your head and will be easy to wear for extended periods of time.

Scarves that are too silky will not stay tied as tightly as a scarf with some cotton or other fabric blend in it. But don't let this be the reason for rejecting a scarf that will enhance a particular outfit; there are ways around this problem. Sometimes fashion has to trump wear-ability!

You will want to have a few square scarves in different sizes as they can be tied quickly and effortlessly. I have a couple of square cotton scarves that I wear when I do my yard work. After I wear them in the hot sun, they are washed easily in the washing machine. Also be sure to apply sunscreen on your face and hands and wear a sun hat over the scarf because if you are on chemo you are more sensitive to the sun.

Some women like to wear a soft cotton cap over their head. This will provide additional warmth as well as a little bit more padding under your scarf, which you may prefer.

There is no one answer as to which style of scarf is the best to use. My Mother had many beautiful, expensive scarves that I wanted to wear on occasion. These large silk square designer scarves were vibrant, but no matter how I tried, I was never satisfied with the wearability of these beautiful scarves on my head. So remember, you may not be able to use every scarf that you love.

Chapter Three

The Triangle Fold

❧

This is probably the easiest and most well-known way to tie a scarf. You simply take a square scarf and fold it in half diagonally. You center the fold over the center of your forehead and bring the ends around to the back of your head and tie it in a knot.

This can be done with a square scarf of just about any size…from miniscule to really large. Medium-sized cotton bandana scarves are comfortable to wear (with or without a hat) while working in the yard.

If the ends of the scarf are long enough, you may also tie it into a bow. When tied in a bow, you are then able to take the "bows" and spread them apart and fluff them out. This creates the effect of having a puff or a flower at the back of your head, softens the effect of the scarf, and makes a very pretty fashion statement.

A slight variation is to lift up some of the extra fabric in the scarf and let a little bit of it "poof" over the bow. This slightly changes the profile appearance, making it appear a little softer.

For variation, the scarf may be tied on the side of your head instead of at the back. This is very pretty with a longer scarf as the tails of the scarf will hang down to the side of your face and softly frame it. You can even pretend that you have braids pulled to one side of your head!

You will be amazed how the slightest adjustment can make an immense difference in how the scarf appears, which will also make a wonderful difference in how you feel.

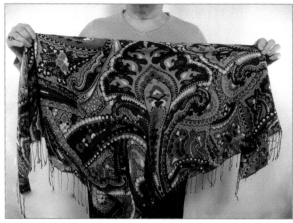

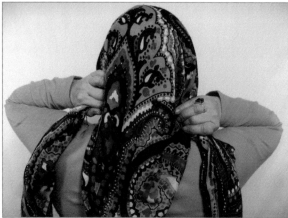

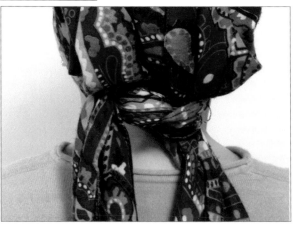

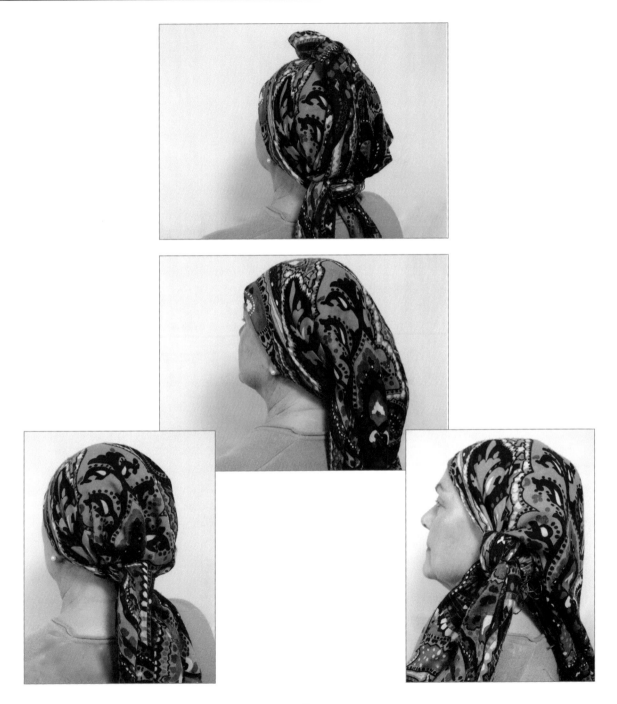

Chapter Four

Turbans

A turban is my favorite way to tie my scarves. It appears more complicated than it actually is, but after a little practice, you'll be able to tie one easily.

The longer rectangular scarves are made for this style. And, personally, I think that the longer they are, the more interesting are the combinations achieved with them. Many of these scarves have tassels on the ends and you want to be sure to use this design element to your advantage.

After you review the suggestions given in Chapter Two on scarf shopping, remember that you want to be sure your scarf coordinates with and enhances the overall effect of your outfit.

You will want to put on a little make-up, paying particular attention to your eyes. If your eyelashes are gone ~ smudge a little eyeliner on your upper eyelid and almost no one will notice the difference. Make sure that your eyebrows extend to their normal length ~ with a little help, of course! You will not only look better, but you will feel better also.

Now, let's tie one on!

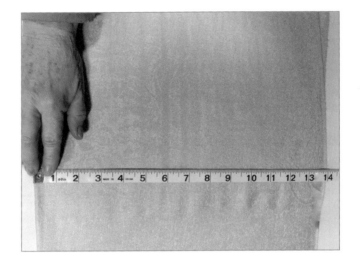

a) Start by folding the scarf lengthwise so that it is about 14 inches wide. You want it to be just wide enough to cover your head from the forehead to the nape of your neck. Depending on the size of your head, you may need to fold your scarf anywhere from 13" to 16". Those of you with a small head may need to fold your scarf to 13 inches. After a few tries, you will be able to fold your scarf to the correct dimension for yourself without even measuring.

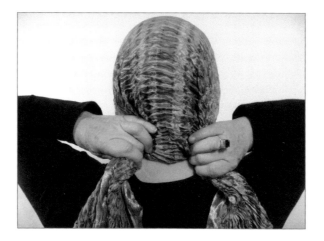

b) Drape the scarf over your head, centering it lengthwise on your forehead. Then grasp both ends and pull them firmly around to the back of your head. You have now covered your entire head smoothly with your scarf and the ends are at the back of your head.

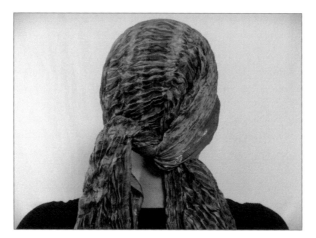

c) At this point it is important to pull your scarf tight and tie it tightly. This is the secret to making your turban look good so it stays securely on your head for many hours.

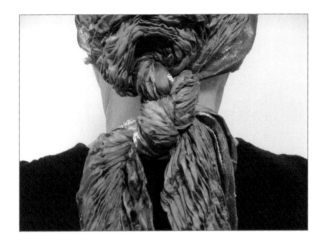

At this time you do one of three things:
1) Tie it once.
2) Tie it in a double knot or even a triple knot.
3) Or just cross the ends from one side to the other, switching the ends in your hands.

What you decide to do will vary depending on your scarf's fabric, the length of your scarf, and the mood that you want to achieve. I'll explain how you make this decision a little later.

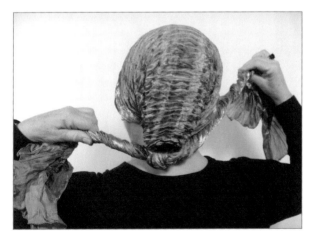

d) This next step is important and may take a little practice. Start twisting both ends of the scarf. If you start twisting each side in a downward direction, you will find that it will sit over your ears better.

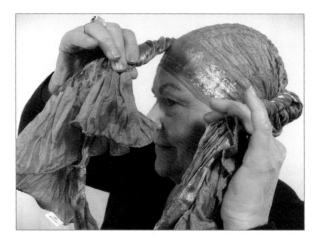

e) As you twist the ends, wrap the scarf around your head. The tighter you twist the scarf, the more fabric will be used up. A looser twist will use less fabric. I'll explain the reason for this later also. Continue to wrap the ends around your head tightly, crossing the "rolls" over each other at least once. This makes your turban more interesting.

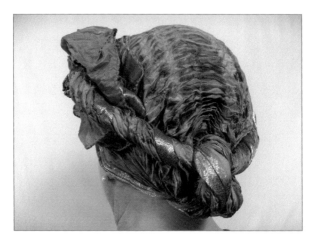

f) Then continue wrapping the ends around your head until you can bring them together and tie them securely. Again, you may need to tie another knot (or two) to use up the extra fabric.

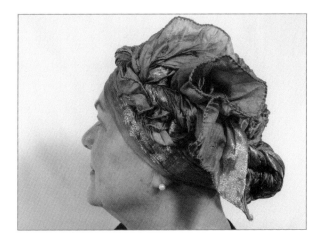

Sometimes you may end up tying your scarf at the back of your head, sometimes at the side, sometimes at the front. I particularly like the way a turban looks when it is tied on the side; with the tassels hanging down it can be quite elegant as well as fun and interesting. Babies and little girls find this look especially irresistible!

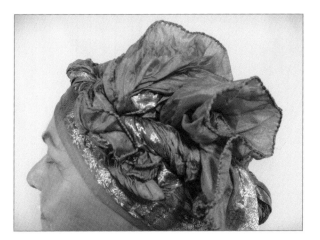

It is also possible to "fluff up" the tied ends of your scarf and have your very own Fascinator! Adding a pin or a flower to your scarf once it is tied allows you to further express your personal sense of fashion. Make the most of this new experience in your life.

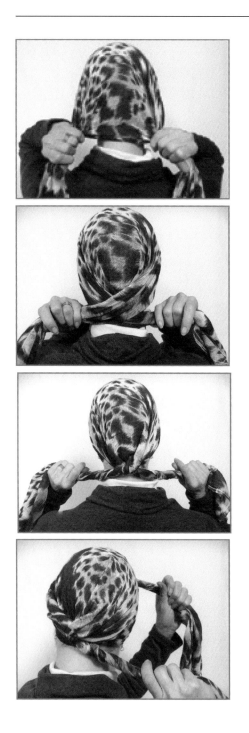

Place & Pull

Cross & Tie

Twist

Wrap

Cross Rolls

Tie

Intriguing

Beautiful

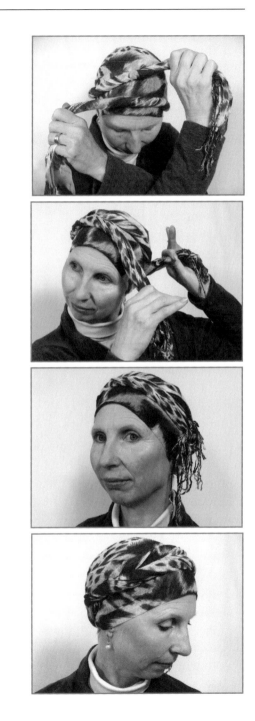

Now for the "later" explanation….

Not all scarves will be the same length, and what may work for one scarf may not work for another. Where you end up tying your turban is important, and with each different scarf you need to have some flexibility in determining just how special your turban will ultimately look. Offsetting the initial placement of your scarf slightly will result in the ends being tied to one side of your head, thus giving a more interesting appearance.

Tying is where you are able to manipulate the length of your scarf somewhat. If your scarf is a little bit too long, you can tie another knot or two at the back of your neck before you start twisting and wrapping it around your head. This cluster of knots presents a very attractive appearance when finished.

The same thing goes for twisting ~ the tighter you twist it, the shorter your scarf will become. And conversely, the looser you twist it, the closer it stays to its original length. These are suggestions that you can employ to manipulate the placement of your final tie, i.e., front, side, back.

Please note that there are some fabrics that look especially beautiful if only slightly twisted; others are prettier when twisted more tightly. This is where your personal creativity comes into play. But remember to pull the scarf tightly around your head in the first step before you tie it at the nape of your neck!

A dramatic style is to layer two scarves, one on top of the other, before placing on your head. A very interesting combination results when you twist the two scarves together and wrap around your head. This is the technique that I created when tying the turban that you see in my author's photo.

It is also possible to carefully remove a tied turban and then put it on the next day, just as you would a hat, with only a few minor adjustments. I would do this when I was feeling especially tired. Most of the time I could get away with not having to retie my scarf and it looked as stylish the second day as it did the first.

Remember that you are learning a new skill and that it may take some time to master these techniques. Please persevere and before long you will be tying your gorgeous scarves expertly and wearing them with beautiful confidence.

8 Steps to a Perfect Turban

1. **PLACE** your scarf on your head

2. **PULL** it tight

3. **TIE** a knot in the back

4. **TWIST** the scarf ends

5. **WRAP** the ends around your head

6. **TIE** the ends together

7. **FLUFF** the ends

8. **SMILE** and **BE CONFIDENT**

Chapter Five

Hats

There are many benefits to wearing a scarf under your hat. It will protect your head in case your hat is scratchy. It will help keep your head warm ~ very important in air conditioning and when traveling on airplanes. And it will help your hat feel more secure. A scarf will also soften the effect of your hat because you will be framing your face with your scarf instead of your hair under your hat. Since you will be coordinating your scarf to your outfit, one hat will suffice for many outfits.

The easy triangle fold is a very nice way to wear your scarf under your pretty hat. You can also use a rectangular scarf under your hat. You will simply want to wrap your head with your scarf and then tie it in a bow at the nape of your neck before putting your hat on your head. This look is especially attractive if you fluff up the bow before you put on your hat.

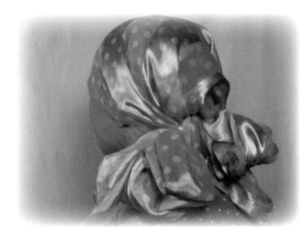

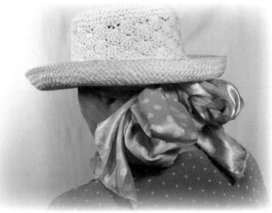

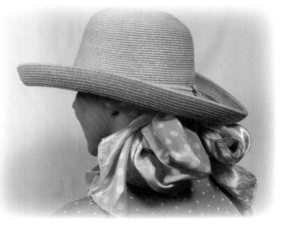

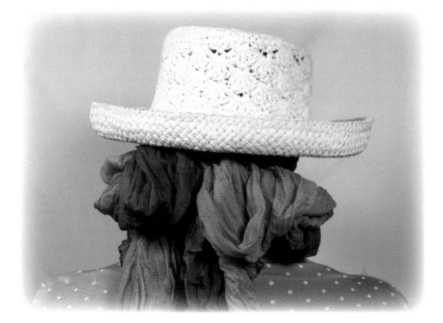

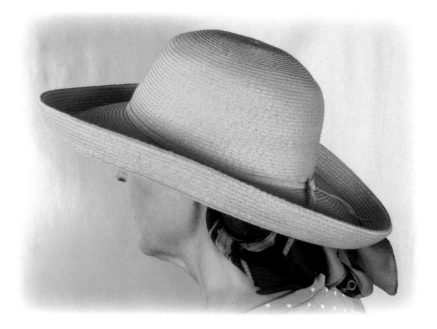

Chapter Six

Sheer Scarves

I do not advocate wearing sheer scarves for several reasons. They are usually made of slippery fabric and therefore do not stay tied securely. But the most important reason is that they do not cover your bald head well enough, and so you must use two scarves.

It is possible to wear a little cap under a sheer scarf, but then the scarf may slip off of the cap, or the cap may slip on your head. Another possibility is to layer the sheer scarf over a solid one before placing on your head.

I have two beautiful pink scarves. They are very sheer, but they were the only pink scarves that I had, and I needed to wear pink to go with my outfit on a particular day. So I put the two scarves together and tied them into one turban. It took a little bit of time and I had to manipulate them because one was considerably shorter than the other, but the end effect was really delightful.

Just persist and you'll be able to come up with a style that will reflect your individual personality and please you.

How to Make a Scarf Rosette...

There is a very simple way to make a beautiful rosette out of the ends of your scarf. The technique is quite simple and actually works best with a sheer or lightweight scarf as opposed to one that is thicker and has more body to it.

1. Tie the scarf on the side of your head ~ allowing the ends to hang down.

2. Hold the ends together and start twisting them.

3. Keep twisting them until the ends are tightly twisted and it looks sort of like a rope.

4. Wrap the "rope" around the knot in a spiral.

5. Tuck the ends in and...

6. Voila! A scarf rosette!

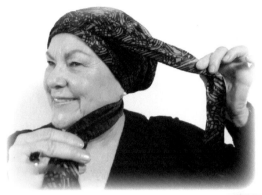

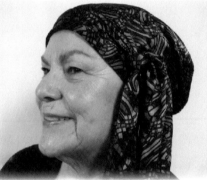

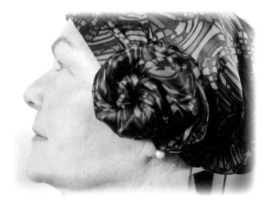

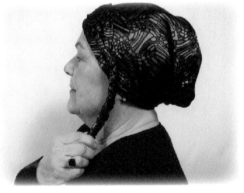

Chapter Seven

After Your Hair Grows Back

When your hair starts growing back in, you will be very excited to see your new look. If your hair loss was due to chemotherapy, your new hair may be an entirely different color and texture. A vibrant red or distinctive grey are often unexpected but common colors to be showing up in this new hair growth. And just as chemotherapy will kill all the cancer in your body, it may also literally curl your hair. My dark blond straight hair came in a beautiful dark grey color and as soft and curly cute as a little poodle puppy! No matter if you love or hate your new hair, it usually will return to your normal shade and texture within the year, or so I've been told. The curls do usually grow out within six months, so if curls are new to you, enjoy them while you have them because they probably will go away sooner than you would like.

Now that you have hair, what will you do with your new wardrobe of beautiful scarves that have served you so well over the last many months? You have several choices. You may choose to keep them in case they might be needed again; you may choose to donate them to your local cancer treatment center or local cancer society for reuse by another devastated woman; or you may choose to keep them and wear them as an accessory.

If you choose to wear your scarves as an accessory in your wardrobe, I have pictured a few ways they can be styled. You should consider gently cleaning the scarves that you have worn the most. And don't forget to press the wrinkles out of the ones you plan to wear. You want to continue looking your best. Enjoy!

Chapter Eight

Styling

❧

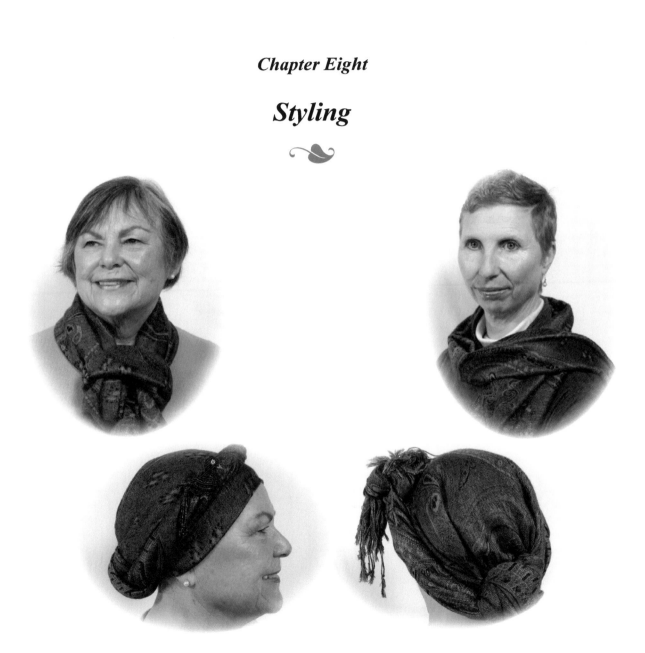

Styling

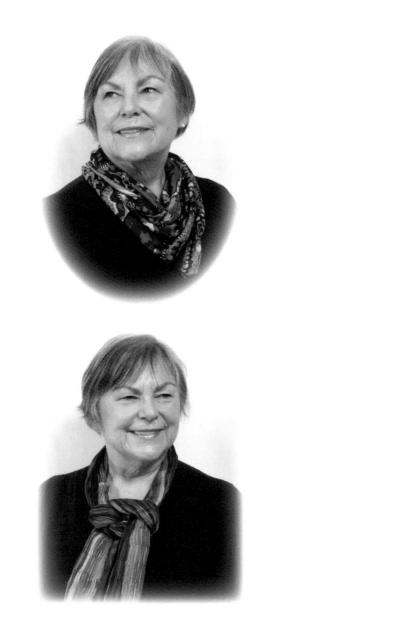

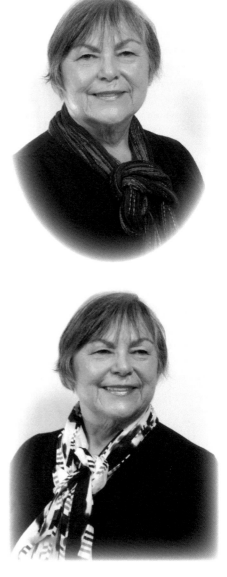

Styling

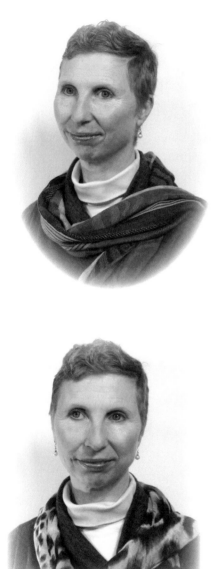
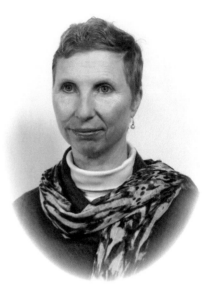
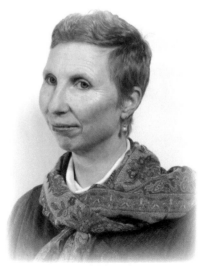

Styling

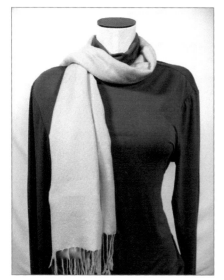

Sophisticate

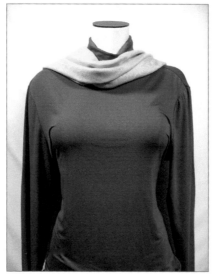

Diana

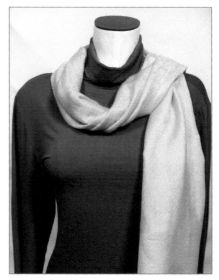

Sophisticate

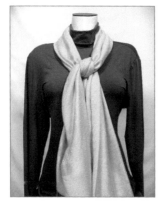

Sadie

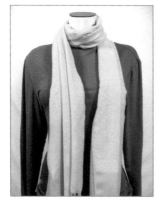

Mercedes

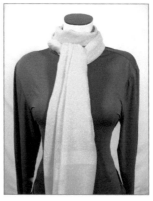

Ascot

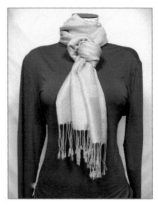

Why Knot

Styling

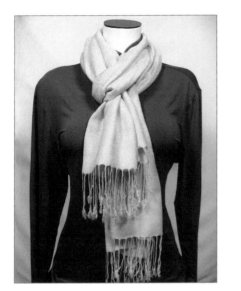

Portland

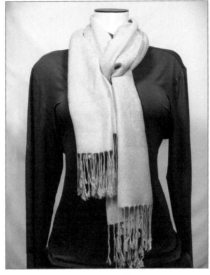

Portlandia

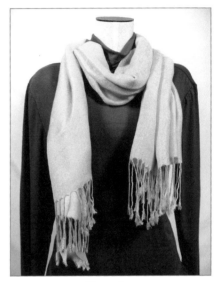

Seattle

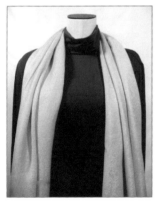

Let It Be

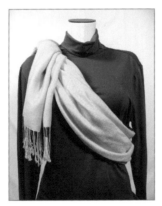

Heather

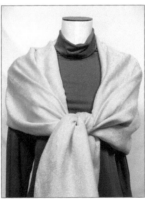

European

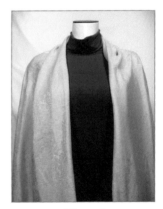

Shawl

Chapter Nine

Recap

Here are some things for you to remember as you travel this new phase in your life. Do experiment with different patterns and lengths of scarves to discover the looks you like the best and what looks the best on you.

Scarves are an accessory ~ so remember to look for scarves that go with, not necessarily match, your outfit.

Always keep your eyes open when shopping. One never knows when you may find the perfect scarf for which you have been searching.

Be patient ~ it may take a little practice to become proficient at wrapping, twisting and tying your scarves. Remember, you are learning a new skill set and that may take a little bit of time. Just persevere and you will soon become very adept at tying one on!

Many organizations have scarves that have been donated to them by other patients. A good place to start looking for resources in your area would be your local cancer center, hospital, or cancer society.

And most of all…if you like the way you look, you will exude confidence and everyone who looks at you will see that confidence and will also admire the way you look.

Be creative! Portland Firefly hopes that this phase in your life is short-lived and that your hair will be growing in soon! Good luck!

Chapter Ten

No Hair ~ No Problem

Some Good Things about Having No Hair

1. My bathroom sink looks much neater without the hairdryer, curling iron, brushes and combs all over!

2. Think of the money I'll save on shampoo, mousse, conditioners and hairspray!

3. It takes me way less time to get ready in the morning!

4. I now have an excuse to wear adorable hats and scarves! And if people look at me weird ~ too bad for them!

5. I like hats ~ I'll probably get tired of wearing them, but right now, I like my turban style scarf! "It brings out my eyes!"

6. I'll probably get fewer colds because my head will always be covered and it won't get cold!

7. I won't have to waste time at the beauty shop!

8. Think of the money I'll save on hair coloring products!

9. I'll save more money on haircuts!

10. I can change my hairstyle on a whim with just a different wig!

11. I won't need to shave my legs!

12. No need for a painful bikini wax!

13. My drains won't get clogged with hair!

14. I can ride in a convertible and my hair won't get messed up!

15. I won't have a bad hair day!

Chapter Eleven

Biographies

Andrew Creasy ~ Photographer

A talented and artistic young man, Andrew Creasy knew his passion was in visual arts at a young age. In June 2010, Andrew earned a BA in Media Arts with a concentration in Film Production and a minor in Business Administration, thus becoming the first Film Production graduate in Eastern Oregon University history. Andrew keeps active in the film industry, working on various Portland productions on his way to one day becoming a Hollywood cinematographer and director.

"I am thrilled to be able to participate in this worthwhile project."

Brenda Payne McGowan ~ Model

Brenda is a retired Pediatric Nurse who is widowed and lives on a small farm in the lower Willamette Valley. She enjoys fly-fishing, camping, reading, the symphony, opera, birding and travel. Nature brings her comfort, solitude and contentment. She is surrounded by two step children, their spouses, six grandchildren and a loving and supportive group of cherished friends.

She was diagnosed with Stage IIIC Ovarian Cancer in January, 2009. She wore scarves and hats, which added color and gave her an air of confidence during her recovery.

"I remain positive. I savor each day…Each day is a GIFT."

Marcy Westerling ~ Model

Marcy Westerling is a community organizer who has been based in Oregon for over 25 years. She is in a long-term relationship with her best friend and organizing colleague. They share a passion for growing their own foods and making the world a more just place.

She was diagnosed with Stage IV Ovarian Cancer just after her 51st birthday in April, 2010. After completing front line treatment, she continues to work, albeit at a calmer pace and scale.

"I am truly learning how to live and thrive one day at a time."

Signs and Symptoms of Ovarian Cancer

Ovarian cancer is difficult to detect, especially in the early stages. This is partly due to the fact that ovaries, two small almond-shaped organs, one on each side of the uterus, are deep within the abdominal cavity. In addition, we as women tend to minimize our physical ailments, explain them away, and do not give them the importance they deserve. The symptoms of ovarian cancer are vague and mimic other illnesses, which is why ovarian cancer is most often misdiagnosed. These are some of the reasons that, when it is finally diagnosed, ovarian cancer has progressed to late stage and the survival rate is greatly diminished.

Potential Signs and Symptoms of Ovarian Cancer

- Abdominal pressure, fullness, swelling or bloating
- Urinary urgency
- Pelvic discomfort or pain
- Persistent indigestion, gas or nausea
- Unexplained changes in bowel habits, such as constipation or diarrhea
- Changes in bladder habits, including a frequent need to urinate
- Loss of appetite or quickly feeling full
- Increased abdominal girth or clothes fitting tighter around your waist
- Pain during intercourse
- A persistent lack of energy which is often described as fatigue
- Low back pain
- Changes in menstruation

If these symptoms persist for more than two weeks, you should ask your physician for a pelvic and a rectal examination. Additional evaluation may include a transvaginal ultrasound, a blood test called the CA-125, a CT scan or an X-ray.

When symptoms are persistent, that is, when they do not resolve with normal interventions (like diet change, exercise, laxatives, and rest), it is imperative for a woman to see her doctor. Persistence of symptoms is a key component in diagnosing ovarian cancer. Because the signs and symptoms of ovarian cancer have been described as vague, only about 19% of ovarian cancer is found in the early stages. Symptoms typically occur in advanced stages when tumor growth creates pressure on the bladder and the rectum and fluid begins to form. Primary Peritoneal Carcinoma is a rare type of ovarian cancer that occurs in women who have had a partial or complete hysterectomy. This is why general awareness of ovarian cancer symptoms is a must for every woman.

Organizations Supporting Ovarian Cancer Awareness, Education, Advocacy and Research

Ovarian Cancer Alliance of Oregon and Southwest Washington
(OCAOSW)
www.ovariancancerosw.org

Sherry Hildreth Ovarian Cancer Foundation
(SHOC)
www.shocfoundation.org

Ovarian Cancer National Alliance
(OCNA)
www.ovariancancer.org

National Ovarian Cancer Coalition
(NOCC)
www.ovarian.org

Look Good, Feel Better
www.lookgoodfeelbetter.org
1-800-395-5665

American Cancer Society (ACS)
www.cancer.org

The cover on this book is teal because teal is the color for ovarian cancer.
A portion of the proceeds of this book will support ovarian cancer
awareness, education, advocacy and research.

He has sent me to bind up the brokenhearted…
To comfort all who mourn…
To bestow on them a crown of beauty instead of ashes,
The oil of gladness instead of mourning,
And a garment of praise instead of a spirit of despair.

Isaiah 61:1-3

Additional copies of *TIE ONE ON* are available through

http://xulonpress.com/bookstore
1-866-909-BOOK
1-866-909-2665

Barnes & Noble

Google Books

Amazon.com

eBook

and

Espresso Book Machine

A special hard-cover edition for office waiting rooms
with **OFFICE COPY ~ DO NOT REMOVE** on the cover
is available by special order through
http://xulonpress.com/bookstore
1-866-909-BOOK
1-866-909-2665

CPSIA information can be obtained
at www.ICGtesting.com
Printed in the USA
240389LV00001B